First Steps through the Menopause

Catherine Francis

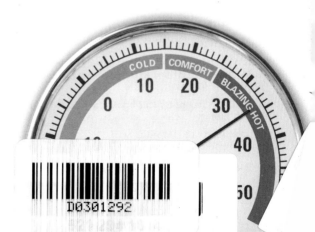

COLD COMFORT BLAZING HOT

0 10 20 30 40 50

D0301292

All advice given is for information only and should not be treated as a substitute for qualified medical advice.

Copyright © 2012 Catherine Francis
This edition copyright © 2012 Lion Hudson

The author asserts the moral right to be identified as the author of this work

A Lion Book
an imprint of
Lion Hudson plc
Wilkinson House, Jordan Hill Road,
Oxford OX2 8DR, England
www.lionhudson.com
ISBN 978 0 7459 5557 5 (print)
ISBN 978 0 7459 5705 0 (e-pub)
ISBN 978 0 7459 5704 3 (Kindle)

Distributed by:
UK: Marston Book Services, PO Box 269, Abingdon,
Oxon, OX14 4YN
USA: Trafalgar Square Publishing, 814 N. Franklin Street,
Chicago, IL 60610
USA Christian Market: Kregel Publications, PO Box 2607,
Grand Rapids, MI 49501

First edition 2012
10 9 8 7 6 5 4 3 2 1 0

All rights reserved

This book has been printed on paper and board independently certified as having been produced from sustainable forests.

A catalogue record for this book is available from the British Library

Typeset in 10/12 ITC Stone Serif
Printed and bound in Malta

Contents

Introduction

The menopause used to be referred to in mysterious terms and hushed tones: "She's going through The Change" or "She's turning St Catherine's corner." Even now, the menopause is often seen as something strange and unpleasant to be dreaded – an event that heralds the end of a woman's life as she knows it.

However, the menopause is a perfectly natural transition in the life of every female, and not something to be afraid of. Understanding what's happening in your body, and what physical, mental, and emotional effects you may experience, will help to ease the anxiety or fear of what you are (or may soon be) going through.

Knowledge is power

In this book, you'll learn about the different ways of tackling the physical symptoms that often come with the menopause – through medical means and by natural and alternative methods. You'll discover how hormonal changes may affect you mentally and emotionally, and how you can stay on an even keel. You'll also find out how to deal with changes in your sex life – the one area many women are too embarrassed to ask their doctor about.

You'll learn how to stay looking and feeling good as your body, skin, and hair change with your fluctuating hormones. You'll also discover how to protect yourself from conditions such as osteoporosis and heart disease, which become more of a risk after the menopause, so you can continue enjoying life into old age.

There are also lots of stories from real women, who share what they've experienced and what worked for them.

Take control of your body

Learning how to manage your symptoms will help you stay healthy and happy throughout the menopause and beyond. Many women even come to see this time as a gateway to an exciting new phase of their lives, with more freedom and independence to do the things they want.

After all, women today can expect to live a third or more of their lives post-menopause, and you want to make the most of it, don't you? Well, here's where to start – by taking control of your body and your health.

1

What is the menopause?

The menopause is sometimes described as the reversal of puberty. Both processes are caused by major hormonal changes within your body. Puberty kick-starts sexual development, menstruation, and the beginning of the reproductive phase of your life. The menopause does the opposite – it brings about the end of ovulation and your periods, after which you're no longer able to conceive.

Technically, the menopause is your last menstrual period. However, because periods tend to be irregular during this time, medics usually pinpoint the menopause at twelve months after your final period.

The few years running up to your last period, when you may experience some of the symptoms described in this chapter, is officially known as the "perimenopause". The stage after your last period, when you may continue to experience symptoms for several years, is "post-menopause". However, most people use the term "menopause" fairly loosely to describe all three stages.

The menopause usually occurs between the ages of 45 and 55, with the average age being 52. However, it can be considerably later – up to the age of 60. Before the age of 40, it's classed as a "premature menopause" (you can read more about that in Chapter 9).

Mythbuster

The menopause is a medical condition.
The menopause isn't an illness or disorder requiring medical treatment. It's a perfectly natural stage in every woman's life, and many people sail through it without any problems. However, some of the symptoms caused by your hormones being in flux can be debilitating, and medical treatments or self-help measures can alleviate them. The menopause also increases your risk of other serious health problems, such as osteoporosis (brittle bones). You'll learn how to lower those risks in Chapter 8.

What people say...
I started experiencing menopausal symptoms at 41. My periods stopped at 46, and I'm nearly through it now. Some of what you read about the menopause is so depressing, especially concerning things like your sex life. However, my only real symptom has been hot flushes, which have been quite manageable. It's great not having periods or having to worry about pregnancy any more. And I'm glad to report that my husband and I still enjoy a good sex life.
Sabina, 49

What's happening in your body?

Just as puberty is caused by increasing levels of the female hormones oestrogen and progesterone in your body, the menopause is caused by these hormones declining.

The main hormone at work is oestrogen, which is actually the collective term for three hormones: oestradiol, oestrone, and oestriol. Oestrogen is produced mainly in the ovaries, and in small amounts by the adrenal glands. As well as many other bodily functions, it regulates your menstrual cycle, causing you to have periods and release an egg every month.

As levels of oestrogen in your body slowly drop during your 40s and 50s, your ability to conceive diminishes, and you can experience a variety of symptoms. These can last for up to ten years, but for most women they last between two and six years. Eventually, your ovaries stop producing eggs, your periods stop, and the menopause has occurred.

Diminishing levels of other sex hormones, including progesterone and testosterone (yes, women's bodies produce some "male" hormones too), also play their part in menopausal symptoms. However, oestrogen is the main culprit.

Mythbuster

My mother had a tough menopause, so I will too.
The age at which your mother had her menopause can give an indication as to when you're likely to have yours. However, when it comes to symptoms, there's no evidence of a genetic link. Just because your mother had a difficult time, it doesn't mean you will. Every woman's experience is different.

What symptoms might you experience?

The main sign that your menopause is approaching is that your periods become further apart or irregular. They may also be lighter and shorter, or they may be heavier and last longer – everyone is different. In some women, periods stop altogether without warning. However, you should remember that heavy or irregular periods can also be an indicator of medical conditions such as fibroids or polyps, so you should always mention them to your doctor.

As well as irregular periods, there are a number of other symptoms you may experience. Don't panic – you're unlikely to have all of them.

Hot flushes

Hot flushes are one of the most common symptoms of the menopause, experienced by three out of four women. They involve feeling hot and sweaty, usually in your upper body, often starting in your face, neck, or chest. They usually last for a few minutes, and are sometimes followed by feeling cold. Your skin may go red and patchy, and some women experience a "crawling" sensation on the skin. You may also have palpitations (increased heart rate). Hot flushes can occur several times a day.

Night sweats

These are hot flushes that occur at night, often with severe sweating that can leave your nightwear and bedclothes drenched.

Mood swings

These include tearfulness, irritability, anxiety, panic attacks, and depression. You're more likely to experience emotional changes if you've had similar symptoms with pre-menstrual syndrome (PMS). Depression and anxiety can be made worse by oestrogen deficiency – but don't discount the events or stresses in your life that may be contributing to your emotional distress.

Vaginal dryness
This is caused by the body producing less natural lubricant and by the thinning of the vaginal walls, which can also lead to loss of elasticity. It's experienced by around a third of women after the menopause, and it can make sex uncomfortable or painful. However, there are ways around this, which you can read more about in Chapter 5. Dryness can also lead to itching and general discomfort in the vulval area.

Lower libido
As oestrogen and other sex hormones drop, this can lead to a decrease in sexual desire (not helped by the discomfort of vaginal dryness). However, some women enjoy sex more after the menopause, so don't assume it's the end of your sex life.

Interrupted sleep
Lower levels of oestrogen can affect the quality of your sleep and lead to insomnia. Night sweats can also disturb your sleep (and your partner's), as can depression and anxiety.

Poor concentration and memory
Oestrogen contributes to the functioning of brain cells, so a drop in oestrogen may result in lower concentration

levels and memory lapses. This may be made worse by fatigue from disturbed sleep.

Dry skin
Lower levels of oestrogen make it harder for your skin to retain moisture. Skin also becomes thinner with age, which can lead to dryness and itching.

Urinary problems
Around one in six women develops a urinary tract problem during the menopause. Stress incontinence (leaking urine when coughing or laughing) can become an issue, due to thinning of the tissue and loss of elasticity. This can also lead to reduced bladder capacity, which means you may need to pass urine more often. There's also an increased risk of urinary tract infections.

General aches and pains
Lower levels of oestrogen can contribute to joint pains, muscular pains, and headaches.

Mythbuster

Women always go through hell with the menopause.
Most women experience some symptoms during the menopause. However, for many, these are relatively mild – and some feel no effects at all. If you experience unpleasant symptoms, there are plenty of measures you can take to reduce or eliminate them. So don't be discouraged – read on to learn how you can start taking control of your body.

How is the menopause diagnosed?

Your doctor will be able to confirm that you're probably approaching the menopause, based on your age, the pattern of your periods, and your symptoms. However, it's not always possible to be certain, especially if you're taking the contraceptive pill or other hormonal treatments. There's no definitive medical test for the menopause. Measuring the levels of follicle-stimulating hormone (FSH) in your blood can help to confirm a diagnosis, as FSH rises in women who are approaching the menopause. However, the test isn't always accurate and isn't enough on its own to confirm that you're menopausal.

What people say...
I started missing a few periods when I was 45, and when I did have them, my PMS was worse than before. After eight months, I started having hot flushes. My face and chest go red and feel like they're on fire – it's a bit embarrassing when I'm at work, although the women of my age are very supportive of each other. I spoke to my doctor and decided not to go down the HRT route yet, although I'm keeping an open mind about it. Improving my diet and exercising more have helped my symptoms somewhat. Having an understanding husband helps too.
Phillipa, 47

Over to you!

If you're experiencing one or more of the symptoms described in this chapter, make an appointment with your doctor. Many of these symptoms can have other medical causes, such as fibroids, so it's best to get them checked out. Alternatively, your doctor may be able to confirm that you're probably approaching the menopause, and you can discuss your options. However, you may want to read the next few chapters first, so you're informed about the options available to you and know what to ask.

2

Hormone replacement therapy (HRT)

The most common medical treatment offered to alleviate unpleasant menopausal symptoms is hormone replacement therapy (HRT). This boosts your levels of the female hormones your body is naturally producing less of.

HRT can be very effective at relieving symptoms caused by oestrogen deficiency, such as hot flushes, vaginal dryness, and sleep disturbances. It can also help protect you against more serious health conditions, such as osteoporosis, particularly in women who've had an early menopause. However, not everyone is suitable for HRT, and there are some risks attached to it, so it's a good idea to consider all the options before making a decision.

How does HRT work?

There are over sixty different types of HRT on the market. Some are oestrogen-only, and some are "combined", containing oestrogen and progestogen (a synthetic replacement for progesterone).

Oestrogen plays an important role in many body functions, so if your natural levels are waning, a replacement can alleviate many unpleasant symptoms. The oestrogen in HRT is usually extracted from plants or from the urine of pregnant horses.

Declining levels of progesterone don't have such a dramatic effect on your body, but progesterone offers protection against cancer of the lining of the womb (the endometrium), so a replacement progestogen is used in some forms of HRT.

There are three main types of HRT:

Continuous combined HRT

This is usually prescribed for women whose periods have stopped. It contains both oestrogen and progestogen, and is taken daily.

Cyclical or sequential HRT

This is usually recommended for women who are having menopausal symptoms but are still having periods. It involves taking oestrogen every day, and progestogen for fourteen days at the end of your cycle. This cycle may last a month or three months (in which case, you'll only have a period every three months).

Oestrogen-only HRT
This is usually recommended for women who've had a total hysterectomy (including removal of the cervix and possibly ovaries), as they are no longer at risk of endometrial cancer. For a partial hysterectomy, where some of the womb lining is still present, combined HRT may offer better protection. Around a fifth of British women have had a hysterectomy by the age of 55.

Mythbuster

HRT will make me fat.
It's common to gain weight around the time of the menopause, but there's no evidence that HRT is the culprit – it would probably happen whether or not you're taking HRT. However, there are lots of things you can do to keep the extra pounds at bay – see Chapter 6 to find out more.

The benefits of HRT
Many women swear by the effects of HRT for giving them a better quality of life. It can dramatically improve symptoms such as hot flushes, vaginal dryness, urinary tract infections, stress incontinence, and mood swings. The benefits usually kick in within a week or two. Many women also find it helps to keep their skin supple and boosts their libido.

HRT can play a small part in reducing your risk of cancers of the colon and rectum. It also helps protect you against osteoporosis, as oestrogen is important for healthy bone growth (you'll learn more about that in Chapter 8).

What people say...

I never thought I'd take HRT – I always thought I'd embrace ageing stoically and surf the changes as they happened. But of course it's not like that, especially when symptoms start earlier than expected – in my case, my early 40s. Sleepless nights, the embarrassment of hot flushes in business meetings, aching joints, being hellishly irritable – it felt like thrashing about with no exit in sight. Going on HRT almost instantly restored me to how I was before. I feel I have my old self back, not this alien body that let me down. Now I'm nervously counting the days until I have to come off the HRT again.
Rhea, 46

The downsides of HRT

Some women experience unpleasant side effects from HRT, especially when they first start taking it. These usually settle down within three months, but if you have any problems, talk to your doctor. He or she may alter your dose, try you on a different type of HRT, or suggest another way of taking it.

The side effects of oestrogen in HRT can include fluid retention and bloating, breast tenderness, nausea, headaches, indigestion, and leg cramps. The side effects of progestogen can include mood swings, depression, and acne. Staying active and eating a healthy, low-fat diet can help to reduce these side effects.

However, every woman is different and you won't necessarily have any negative side effects at all.

Mythbuster

HRT just doesn't suit me.

If you're having unpleasant side effects from HRT, it's worth giving it a few months to see if it settles down. If it doesn't, there are dozens of different types of HRT – and just because one type doesn't suit you, it doesn't mean another won't. If you have any problems or concerns, but you want to persevere with taking HRT as a solution to your symptoms, ask your doctor to help you find the type that works best for you.

What are the risks of HRT?

There have been many news reports and scare stories about HRT raising your risk of hormone-related cancers, such as breast and ovarian cancer, and increasing your likelihood of blood clots and stroke. So what are the facts?

Breast cancer

According to Cancer Research UK, taking HRT very slightly increases your risk of breast cancer – and the longer you take it, the greater the risk. Combined HRT raises your risk more than oestrogen-only HRT. However, within five years of coming off HRT, your risk returns to normal. So if you're taking HRT, it's especially important to practise self-examination and keep up with breast screening.

Endometrial cancer

Taking oestrogen can slightly increase your risk of cancer of the endometrium (womb lining). However, with combined HRT, which includes progestogen, there's no increased risk. If you've had a total hysterectomy (including removal of the cervix), the risk is eliminated, so oestrogen-only HRT may be the best option.

Ovarian cancer
Studies have shown that taking HRT slightly increases your risk of ovarian cancer – and the longer you take it, the greater the risk. Once you stop taking HRT, your risk returns to normal over the next few years.

Strokes, heart attacks, and blood clots
Research has found that HRT slightly increases your risk of abnormal blood clotting and high blood pressure. This, in turn, may slightly elevate your risk of stroke and heart attack, especially if you're already at high risk – for instance, if you smoke or are overweight.

Although all these risks are very low, most doctors recommend a time limit for taking HRT – usually no longer than five years. Most experts agree that if it's used for five years or less, the benefits outweigh the risks.

If you experience any unexpected heavy bleeding, shortness of breath, chest pain, or a swollen, painful leg, you should stop taking your HRT immediately and see a doctor urgently. You should see your doctor at least once a year for a check-up anyway, for as long as you're taking it.

HRT may not be suitable for you if you have a history (or family history) of any of these conditions. You may also be unable to take it if you have liver disease or untreated high blood pressure (although you may be able to start once your blood pressure is under control). You can't take HRT if you're pregnant, and it's rarely prescribed for women over 60.

I can't take HRT, so I'll just have to suffer.
If you're unable to take HRT, your doctor may suggest
other medical treatments to tackle your symptoms.
Antidepressants can help with anxiety and mood
swings, and some types can also help reduce hot flushes.
Clonidine, which was designed to treat high blood
pressure, can also help with hot flushes and night sweats.
Vaginal lubricants can be used to relieve dryness. Tibolone
is a synthetic hormone that acts in a similar way to HRT
(and stops periods). There are also plenty of natural
remedies and lifestyle changes that may help – you'll read
more about them in the next chapter.

What people say...
*When I was 41, I had a minor stroke. I made a full recovery
and went on to have two children, but it meant I wasn't a
suitable candidate for HRT. Also, there's a family history of
ovarian cancer – my mum developed it in her 70s, possibly
connected to the fact that she took HRT for fifteen years (the
dangers weren't realized then). So HRT wasn't an option
for me. Fortunately, I didn't find the menopause a difficult
experience and had few symptoms.*
Lorna, 59

How do you take HRT?
You can start taking HRT once you have menopausal
symptoms. Your doctor will probably start you on a low
dose to minimize any side effects, and you can gradually
build up your dose if you need to. HRT can be taken in a
number of ways, depending on your needs.

Tablets
This is the most common way to take HRT – normally one tablet a day.

Patches
These are stuck on the skin, usually on your back, leg, or bottom. The hormone is absorbed into the blood stream through the skin.

Implants
Small, long-lasting pellets are inserted, under local anaesthetic, under the skin (usually in the buttock, thigh, or tummy), where they slowly release the hormone over a number of months.

Creams, gels, and nasal sprays
These are applied to the skin (or sprayed up the nose) to be absorbed into the blood stream. They're sometimes applied in the vagina to combat specific vaginal problems.

Pessaries or vaginal "rings"
These are inserted into the vagina and are particularly useful for treating vaginal symptoms, if this is your main problem.

When should you stop taking HRT?

Most women stay on HRT for between two and five years, to get them over the worst menopausal symptoms. Your doctor will then probably decrease your dose gradually, rather than stop it immediately. Menopausal symptoms may return once you stop taking HRT, but should pass within a few months. If your symptoms don't ease after that, go back to your doctor.

Over to you!

If you think HRT might be the right option for you, discuss the pros and cons with your doctor. This is particularly important if you're at high risk of hormone-related cancers or blood-clotting conditions (in which case HRT may not be suitable for you), or if you're at risk of osteoporosis (in which case HRT may be beneficial). In these cases, your doctor may refer you to a specialist for further advice. Be ready to experiment to find the right type, dose, and method of taking HRT to suit you.

3

The natural approach

If you're not a suitable candidate for HRT, or you don't want to take hormonal treatments, it doesn't mean you have to resign yourself to putting up with unpleasant symptoms. Many women swear by the power of nutrition to carry them through the menopause. Complementary therapies can also be effective for managing symptoms. Even just a few simple lifestyle changes can help to ease the discomfort.

Eat your way through the menopause

A balanced diet is the foundation of a healthy body and can go a long way towards alleviating symptoms. So keep your diet low in saturated fats, sugar, and salt, which are found mainly in processed foods. Eat plenty of fruits, vegetables, lean proteins, healthy oils, nuts and seeds, and wholemeal carbohydrates. Eat little and often to keep your blood sugar levels steady.

There are some key nutrients that play a particularly important role at this time. The mineral calcium is essential for helping to prevent osteoporosis. You can find it in low-fat dairy products, nuts, and green leafy vegetables such as broccoli, kale, and spring greens. You may want to take a supplement to be on the safe side. For calcium to be absorbed, you also need vitamin D, which your body produces in the presence of sunlight and is also found in fish oils, eggs, brown rice, and lentils. For more on lowering your risk of osteoporosis, see Chapter 8.

Other vitamins and minerals that are important during the menopause include vitamin E (found in wholegrain cereals, nuts, rice, and eggs), which may help to reduce hot flushes and vaginal dryness. Zinc is essential for keeping your immune system in good shape and also helps the body absorb calcium. Zinc is found in eggs, green vegetables, pumpkin seeds, and seafood, but its absorption can be lowered by HRT, so you may want to take a supplement as well. Magnesium (in nuts, seeds, and green leafy vegetables) is also important for bone health, and can help to promote better sleep. Potassium (in bananas) is helpful for healthy blood pressure and water retention.

Essential fatty acids omega-3 and omega-6 can be helpful for many menopausal symptoms, including joint pains, vaginal dryness, bladder infections, and dry skin. They also help to increase your energy and sharpen your mind. You'll find them in linseed (flaxseed) oils, pumpkin seeds, walnuts, and oily fish such as sardines, herring, salmon, and tuna. Evening primrose oil and starflower oil contain other essential fatty acids, such as gamma-linolenic acid, which some women find effective for easing symptoms.

The phytoestrogen factor

Some plant foods contain "natural" oestrogens called phytoestrogens – most significantly, a group known as isoflavones. These can help to boost and balance your natural oestrogen levels and ease common symptoms. Good sources include soya products, lentils, beans, linseed (flaxseed) products, fennel, celery, parsley, and red clover. Japanese women have far fewer menopausal symptoms than women in the West, and it's believed to be because their diets include a lot of soya. You'll find soya in tofu and dairy alternatives such as soya milk and soya yogurt. Soya is also thought to help lower the risk of heart disease and breast cancer, both of which increase after the menopause.

What people say...

My hot flushes became intolerable, I was getting two hours' sleep a night and I felt irritable and angry. I didn't want to take HRT, and all my doctor could offer me was sleeping tablets and Prozac. I consulted a homeopath, and his remedies were amazing – my hot flushes really improved. However, sleep still evaded me, so I turned to naturopathy. I gave up alcohol and began detoxing. I cut out processed sugar, gluten, and dairy, and started eating more raw food, hydrating myself properly, and taking essential fatty acids. I gave up red meat and chicken and now eat more fish and vegetables. I feel and look so much better, and if I start slipping back into my old ways, I really notice the difference.

Jane, 50

Lose the toxins

As with almost every condition known to womankind, menopausal symptoms are worsened by nicotine, alcohol, and caffeine. It's believed that smoking can actually lead to an earlier menopause, and it can certainly make hot flushes worse. It also raises your risk of osteoporosis, heart disease, and cancer – all of which increase after the menopause. Excessive alcohol is dangerous for your heart and increases symptoms such as hot flushes, depression, and disturbed sleep. Drink no more than two units of alcohol a day – ideally less – and have at least one alcohol-free day a week. If you fancy a tipple, choose a small glass of red wine, as in moderation this has cardio-protective qualities. Cut back on tea and coffee, as caffeine can play havoc with your blood sugar levels and hinder the absorption of nutrients.

The power of exercise

Regular exercise has been shown to reduce the severity of almost all menopausal symptoms, from hot flushes to poor memory, low sex drive to depression, and sleep problems to lack of energy. It also helps protect you against heart disease, various cancers, and (if the exercise is weight-bearing) osteoporosis.

It doesn't matter what you do, as long as it's something you enjoy and will stick to – cycling, aerobics, swimming, brisk walking, dancing, martial arts, or any other activity that makes you breathless will do the trick. Aim to exercise for at least thirty minutes, five times a week, and keep it varied so you don't get bored. If you're not used to exercising, start gently and build up your stamina. If you have any health conditions, are very overweight, or haven't exercised for a long time, get the OK from your doctor first.

Don't neglect stretching after exercise, as this will help to keep your joints supple and flexible as you get older.

What people say...
I wasn't a suitable candidate for HRT, so instead I turned to natural solutions. I increased my intake of soya products and took black cohosh. I also bought three horses for my teenage children and myself – riding, grooming, and cleaning them out means I get more exercise than I have since I was 20. Perhaps thanks to that, I had very few menopausal symptoms – maybe two or three hot flushes in total.
Lorna, 59

Learn to relax
Avoiding stress can help to reduce most menopausal symptoms, from hot flushes to sleep disorders to depression. Lowering your stress levels can be as simple as learning to say "no", delegating responsibilities at work and at home, or finding time every day to rest – perhaps enjoy a relaxing bath or a good book, whatever works for you. If you find it hard to switch off, a meditation or relaxation class or CD may give you simple techniques for letting go of anxieties. Massage and aromatherapy can help you unwind. If you have particular concerns on your mind, talking to a counsellor could help.

What people say...

HRT didn't suit me, so I went to see a nutritionist, who put me on a diet to sort out my blood sugar levels. I cut back on sugar and wheat, and gave up caffeine. I also took supplements including essential fatty acids, multivitamins and minerals, and a vitamin B complex. My energy levelled out, my painful stiffness eased, and I felt more like myself again. I now know diet can make all the difference to how you feel.
Martine, 49

Take the alternative

There hasn't been a great deal of research done on how effective complementary therapies are for alleviating menopausal symptoms. However, some studies have shown encouraging results, and many women say they get considerable relief from techniques such as acupuncture, homeopathy, reflexology, and aromatherapy. It's important to see a qualified, fully insured therapist, and check that the treatments they're recommending won't react negatively with any medication you're taking, including HRT. Check with your doctor if you're in doubt.

Herbal preparations are particularly effective for relieving symptoms in many women. Many of these can be bought over the counter, although it's advisable to run them past your doctor first, as herbs can be very potent, with possible side effects. Always choose a reputable brand. Here are the most popular herbal remedies:

- *Agnus castus* – for balancing hormones and easing hot flushes and mood swings

- *Black cohosh* – for hot flushes, night sweats, mood swings, and vaginal dryness

- *Dong quai* – for hot flushes and night sweats

- *Evening primrose oil* – for breast tenderness, hot flushes, mood swings, and joint pain

- *Ginkgo biloba* – for improving memory and concentration

- *Ginseng* – for boosting energy, memory, and concentration

- *Kava kava* – for relaxation and better sleep

- *Passion flower* – for rest and improved sleep

- *Sage* – for hot flushes and night sweats

- *St John's wort* – for depression, sleep problems, and anxiety

- *Valerian* – for anxiety, irritability, and better sleep.

What people say...

I suffered from hot flushes, mood swings, urinary problems, night sweats, and insomnia. I didn't want to take HRT, so I tried herbal remedies instead. A combination of black cohosh, sage, and red clover worked for me, and my symptoms are much milder now. I recommend seeing a qualified medical herbalist, as most doctors don't have much time for herbal remedies. It's worth persevering to find the combination of remedies and doses that works for you.
Antonia, 46

Beat the sweats

The unpleasantness of hot flushes and night sweats can be eased by wearing light clothing made from natural fibres such as cotton or hemp, which allow your skin to breathe and moisture to evaporate. Go for layers you can peel off easily. Keeping your bedroom cool and switching to light cotton bedclothes can also help. Having a separate mattress to your partner means you can get up, move around, and change the bedding more easily without disturbing them. Many women find hot flushes and night sweats are triggered or made worse by spicy foods, caffeine, alcohol, smoking, and stress, so experiment to see what works for you. Exercising regularly and drinking plenty of water can also help.

Over to you!

Don't resign yourself to years of miserable symptoms – if you're proactive about discovering what works for you, you can ease or eliminate many of the unpleasant effects of the menopause. Identify which symptoms bother you the most and make a list of methods you can try to beat them. Plan a new diet and exercise regime to boost your general well-being. If you want to try alternative therapies, consult a qualified, registered practitioner. See the **Useful resources** section at the back of this book for help finding a reputable therapist.

4

All in the mind

The menopause is a physical process, but it can affect your mind as much as your body. As oestrogen levels fall, some women are affected mentally, reporting loss of concentration, memory problems, and difficulty sleeping. Others find their moods are affected – depression, anxiety attacks, and mood swings are all common. However, it's not a given that you'll have any of these symptoms, as many women sail through the menopause with no emotional or psychological effects.

Research shows that women on HRT tend to have better short-term memory and concentration, and quicker reaction times, than those not taking it. They also have fewer emotional symptoms. However, that doesn't mean that if you don't take HRT, your brain is destined to turn to mush and you'll spend your days in a tearful heap. There are plenty of self-help methods to ease the strain.

Mind games

Scientists don't fully understand the relationship between oestrogen and mental performance, but it's believed the hormone contributes to the healthy functioning of nerve cells in the brain by helping to build neural connectors and improve blood flow by dilating blood vessels. Your brain is full of oestrogen receptors, particularly in the areas that deal with memory and mood, so it's not surprising that a drop in the hormone can lead to poor concentration and memory – not helped, of course, by fatigue from disturbed sleep.

Many women feel lethargic and lacking in motivation (although, again, this could be partly due to sleepless nights). "Fuzzy thinking" and a short attention span are common complaints.

Mythbuster

I'm going senile.
If you start missing dates in your diary or forgetting where you've parked the car, you may worry that you're developing dementia or Alzheimer's disease. This can be a particular concern if you've seen older relatives suffer with the condition. However, lack of concentration and memory lapses are very normal during the menopausal years – and they won't last for ever.

What people say...

I've become much more irritable since I've been menopausal. My husband gets on my nerves a lot more! My memory isn't as sharp as it was, either – I often forget people's names, which can be embarrassing, especially when I've known them a long

time. I take ginkgo biloba supplements, which have helped
a bit. Being able to talk and laugh about it with friends also
helps – I feel less like I'm going mad.
Glenda, 51

Feeling moody?

Emotional problems aren't inevitable during the
menopause, but some women experience mood slumps
– partly thanks to those oestrogen receptors in the area
of the brain that deals with emotions. It doesn't help
that as oestrogen drops, so does serotonin – the "feel
good" hormone – leaving you feeling tearful, irritable,
or depressed. Some women also battle anxiety and panic
attacks.

Depression is more common during the perimenopausal
years (before your periods stop). You're more likely to
experience emotional changes if you've had pre-menstrual
syndrome (PMS) or post-natal depression in the past.

Mythbuster

Depression? It's just my hormones...
Emotional changes are partly down to fluctuating
hormones, but don't blame it all on your ovaries. Anyone
would feel irritable or depressed if they were battling
sleep problems, hot flushes, sexual difficulties, or urinary
infections. Don't ignore the influence of genuinely
stressful situations in your life – this is a time when many
women are dealing with empty nest syndrome, caring for
elderly parents, and facing divorce or bereavement. The
menopause itself is a significant life change and can be a

profound experience for some women. Coming to terms with the end of your fertility can be a big deal, especially if you've struggled to have children or longed to have more.

What people say...

I was always a happy, active person, but as my periods became less regular, I felt a dark cloud come over me. There was no particular reason for my depression, other than hormonal changes – although I found myself dwelling more on difficult things that had happened in my childhood. I just couldn't shake it off. However, within days of starting HRT, it felt as if the lights had come back on and my depression lifted. Pampering myself with weekly massages also helps me feel like my old self.
Ingrid, 46

Feed your brain

A healthy, balanced diet, rich in omega oils and phytoestrogens, can go a long way towards relieving mental and emotional symptoms during the menopause. Essential fatty acids omega-3 and omega-6 can boost mental energy. Good sources include pumpkin seeds, walnuts, linseeds (flaxseed), the oils from all of these nuts and seeds, and oily fish such as salmon, tuna, mackerel, and sardines.

B vitamins, in particular folic acid, help to build nerve cells and neural connectors. B vitamins are found in wheatgerm, meat, yeast extract, and enriched cereals. Folic acid is primarily found in green leafy vegetables, such as spinach, kale, and broccoli. Antioxidants – vitamins A, C, E, selenium, and beta-carotene – also help protect the brain cells, and magnesium and potassium can help reduce irritability. If you struggle to get all the nutrients you need in your diet, consider taking a supplement.

Aim to eat plenty of low-GI foods (carbohydrates that break down slowly and release energy steadily), such as wholegrain cereals, porridge oats, and vegetables. This will help stabilize your blood sugar, avoiding the peaks and troughs in energy, alertness, and mood that come from sugary, processed foods. Cutting down on caffeine and alcohol can also help to boost your mood and sharpen your mind.

Get moving

Regular exercise can work wonders for combating mental and emotional symptoms. It boosts your mental agility by increasing blood flow to the brain, and can even lower your risk of dementia in the long term. Getting active also releases feel-good hormones serotonin and endorphins, which help to beat stress and raise your mood. It's proven to help combat depression and anxiety. Plus the more active you are, the more energy you'll have.

Be kind to your mind

Keep your concentration and mood as steady as possible by getting as much rest as you can. You could consider booking yourself a regular massage or aromatherapy session to help you unwind. Keep your brain sharp by stimulating it with quizzes and puzzles, studying, or learning new skills. If memory lapses are proving to be a problem, carry a notebook and make notes and lists to help you remember things.

To improve your mood, do something every day that makes you happy, such as taking a gentle walk, watching a comedy DVD, or meeting up with a friend. There's evidence that spending time with people you love improves your happiness levels more than anything else. Talking, laughing together, and hugging people you care about, or even just stroking a pet, all help to raise your levels of serotonin (the happy hormone), lower cortisol (the stress hormone), and reduce blood pressure.

If situations in your life are causing you stress, try to keep talking about them. This could be with a family member, partner, or friend, or you may feel a professional listening ear would be helpful – ask your doctor what's available. Try to identify sources of anxiety and make a plan for reducing their impact. Learn to be assertive about your needs and to say "no".

If you're struggling with depression, your doctor may prescribe antidepressants to get you through the worst. Alternatively, St John's wort ("nature's Prozac") can be very beneficial. The herb acts on transmitters in the brain to improve your mood, and some studies have found it as effective as antidepressants for mild to moderate depression. Other helpful herbal remedies include valerian for anxiety, and ginkgo biloba and ginseng for memory and concentration. Check with your doctor first, though, as herbs should be treated with caution and don't always mix well with conventional medications. Finally, make sure you get out into the daylight every day, especially during winter, as light levels can affect your mood.

For more on dealing with depression and anxiety, there are two helpful books in this series called *First Steps out of Depression* and *First Steps out of Anxiety* – see the **Useful resources** section at the back of this book.

Counting sheep

Waning oestrogen can lead to insomnia for many women. What's more, of course, your quality of sleep isn't helped by symptoms such as night sweats, bladder problems, anxiety, and depression. Lying awake night after night is frustrating, leaving you exhausted during the day. It can also affect your relationship with your partner if you're unable to settle at night or decide you're more comfortable in a separate bed – or even a separate room.

Sleep solutions

First of all, make sure your bedroom is conducive to good rest – quiet, cool, and dark (use an eye mask if your curtains don't block out enough light). Make sure your bed, pillows, and bedclothes are comfortable.

Avoid drinking tea or coffee for several hours before bedtime. Cut out alcohol in the evenings and don't eat a heavy meal late in the day. Go to bed at the same time every night. Working up a sweat several times a week will help to improve your sleep, making it easier to drop off and wake feeling refreshed, but don't exercise too close to bedtime. Having some wind-down time in the evenings can help – a warm bath, perhaps, or listening to calming music. You may want to try a relaxation or meditation CD to help you switch off.

Many people find lavender scent helps them drop off, so try putting some lavender essential oil on a tissue under your pillow. Herbal remedies valerian, kava kava and passion flower all have mild sedative qualities that can help with insomnia (check with your doctor that they don't clash with any medications you're taking).

If you're anxious about something, talking to a counsellor or friend or keeping a journal may stop the worry keeping you awake at night. If night sweats are the problem, turn to Chapter 3 for help dealing with them.

If you're still struggling with sleeplessness, speak to your doctor, who may prescribe sleeping pills on a temporary basis.

Mythbuster

Separate beds will mean the end of my marriage.
Many couples opt for separate beds or separate rooms during this time, and this can certainly help if your partner is disturbed by you tossing and turning all night. You'll also be less stressed if you can stop worrying about waking them. But separate beds don't have to mean the end of sex or affection. Some couples opt for a double bed with separate mattresses. Some start the night in the same bed, with another bed or room to disappear to when things get uncomfortable. If you make the effort to stay connected, separate beds could save your marriage, not end it!

What people say...

I felt dreadful during the menopause – my energy levels plummeted and my sleep patterns were terrible. HRT made me feel worse and I plunged into a deep, dark pit. I had a lively six-year-old daughter to look after, and I was scared I wouldn't cope. A nutritionist put me on a diet and regime of supplements aimed at sorting out my blood sugar balance. I gave up caffeine and took essential fatty acids and a vitamin B complex to boost my mood. Within weeks, I felt more like myself, with renewed energy. My sleep is less interrupted too, helped by a new pillow that moulds to the shape of my neck, so I'm not constantly waking up to fluff and turn my pillow.
Martine, 49

Over to you!

If you're struggling with depression and mood swings, don't suffer in silence. Take a serious look at your lifestyle and see where you can improve your diet, exercise, and daily life to reduce your stress levels and take better care of yourself. Keep talking to friends and family, and ask for their support and understanding if you're not feeling yourself. If depression is seriously affecting your life, book an appointment with your doctor to discuss counselling, HRT, or a temporary course of antidepressants.

5

Sex and relationships

The menopause can have a dramatic impact on your sex life. Many women find their libido (sex drive) wanes. Vaginal dryness is another common complaint, making sex less comfortable. And if you're taking HRT, this may affect the contraceptives you can use. Naturally, these problems can all have a major effect on your marriage or relationship – as can the emotional changes many women experience at this time.

Losing the passion
You may find you become less interested in sex during and after the menopause, and when you're making love with your partner, it may take you longer to become aroused. This is partly due to lower levels of androgens (male hormones, such as testosterone) being produced by your ovaries. If you've had a hysterectomy including the removal of your ovaries, the resulting drop in androgens is

more dramatic and can have an even more marked effect on your libido.

However, sex drive isn't all about hormones. Dealing with symptoms such as hot flushes, mood swings, and fatigue from sleepless nights can understandably mean you have less energy and interest in sex. Meanwhile, night sweats and sleep disturbances mean many couples end up sleeping in separate beds, which doesn't do much for your sex life unless you make the effort to connect at other times.

HRT can help, and other medications such as tibolone and testosterone implants are sometimes offered to post-menopausal women to boost libido. However, exercising regularly, losing weight (if you're overweight), finding time to relax, not smoking, and not drinking too much alcohol have all been shown to improve your sex drive and increase orgasmic potential. Eating well and taking extra zinc and B vitamins may also help.

Low self-esteem can also lead to a lack of interest in sex, and many women's self-image takes a battering during the menopause. You'll have more confidence if you look and feel your best. Turn to Chapters 6 and 7 for advice on staying slim and making the most of your natural beauty.

Mythbuster

All women go off sex after the menopause.
A study by Masters and Johnson[1] found many women remain sexually active well into old age, with no decline in orgasmic potential after the menopause. Some women

---

1. *Sex and Aging: Expectations and Reality* (1986). This finding has been confirmed by subsequent research.

even find their libido increases and they become more orgasmic, possibly because their levels of testosterone become proportionally higher as oestrogen wanes. The end of periods, no concerns about pregnancy, and more privacy after children leave home can all help to give your sexual relationship a new lease of life.

What people say...
Although I still found my husband attractive, I lost interest in sex. How much was to do with hormones, and how much to do with having no sleep thanks to insomnia and night sweats, I'll never know. Certainly I was exhausted just trying to hold down my job and look after two children – sex was the last thing on my mind. My husband was very understanding, but he was relieved when I went on HRT and things returned to normal.
Ruby, 47

Vaginal dryness
Vaginal dryness is experienced by at least a third of women after the menopause. Declining oestrogen levels mean your body tends to produce less natural lubricant. The vaginal walls can also become thinner and more fragile, with less elasticity; and the conditions in the vagina become less acidic and more alkaline, making it more prone to soreness and infection. All this conspires to make sex less comfortable or even painful (known as dyspareunia). Collectively known as vaginal atrophy, these symptoms can develop up to ten years after your last period. Dryness can also lead to general itching and vulval discomfort.

For many women, the solution is as simple as using an over-the-counter sexual lubricant, and taking a more gentle approach to lovemaking. However, if the pain is severe and persistent, you should speak to your doctor.

HRT can dramatically improve vaginal problems, and if this is your only symptom, your doctor may offer you oestrogen cream, gel, or pessaries to be inserted directly into the vagina. These are generally very effective and have the advantage of raising localized hormone levels without affecting your whole body. However, oestrogen creams and gels should not be used as a lubricant during sex, as your partner can absorb the oestrogen through his skin, leading to potential problems.

What people say...

Lovemaking has always been an important part of our thirty-year marriage. During the menopause, my desire to make love wasn't any less, but it became more difficult due to vaginal dryness. The discomfort put me off wanting to try, and my husband was terribly upset that it was painful for me. Now we use a lubricant, which I buy online to avoid embarrassment. It can interrupt the flow of our lovemaking a bit, but we're still able to enjoy it.
Sabina, 49

Irritations and infections

Some women become more prone to lower urinary tract infections (UTIs), such as cystitis, during and after the menopause. This is due to thinning of the tissues in the urethral passage. Penetrative sex may be more likely to cause urinary irritation and increase the risk of UTIs. Because of changes in the alkaline/acid balance in the vagina, there's also an increased risk of bacterial infections – and of these passing to the urinary tract.

Be vigilant about hygiene, but avoid perfumed products, douches, or scrubs. Drinking lots of water and cranberry juice can help to lower your likelihood of a UTI. If you start needing to pass urine more frequently, or it's difficult or painful when you do, see your doctor immediately.

Sex and long-term illness

Disability or becoming less flexible as a result of conditions such as arthritis is likely to affect your sex life. Illnesses such as diabetes and kidney disease can take their toll too, as can certain medications, such as those for high blood pressure, depression, and sleeping problems. Men can also start facing sexual problems in mid-life, such as erectile dysfunction. However, none of this has to spell the end of passion. It may simply mean adapting your sex life to suit you and your partner's changing bodies. You may both require more foreplay and massage to become aroused, and penetrative sex may become a less important feature of your sensual play.

Contraception and the menopause

Don't be fooled into thinking that because you're in your 40s and your periods are slowing down, you won't get pregnant. Women can and do get pregnant in their late 40s and 50s, throughout their perimenopausal years. What's more, as your menstrual cycle becomes less regular, your "fertile" times become unpredictable.

Medics advise that you keep using contraceptives for two years after your last period if you're under 50, and for a year after your last period after the age of 50. However, some forms of contraception (such as progestogen-based methods) may mean you only have occasional periods, or none at all; and some forms of HRT and the contraceptive pill cause you to continue having monthly or three-monthly bleeds for as long as you're taking them. Both of these make it hard to know when you've passed the stage of getting pregnant. Your doctor may recommend a blood test to get a clearer idea of your fertility.

If you're taking HRT, your doctor may advise you to use a non-hormonal or progestogen-only form of contraception, which won't interact with the hormones in your HRT. There are various methods available, including condoms, diaphragm, IUD (intra-uterine device, sometimes called a coil), and the progestogen-only pill. Sterilization (male and female) is also a popular choice for couples whose families are complete.

Mythbuster

I can't get pregnant if I'm taking HRT.
The hormones in HRT are different from the ones used in the contraceptive pill, and HRT won't stop you getting pregnant. So it's essential to continue using contraceptives while you're on HRT, until you're certain you're no longer at risk of pregnancy.

The menopause and your relationship
It's not just changes in your sex life that can affect your marriage or relationship during this time. If you're exhausted thanks to sleepless nights, being driven mad by hot flushes, and battling mood swings and depression, it's hardly surprising if you take your irritation out on

your partner – especially if he doesn't seem supportive or understanding. Meanwhile, he may not be fully aware of what you're going through, and why it should affect your relationship.

Add in the practical stresses you may be facing at this time – children flying the nest (or coming back), caring for elderly parents, and so on – and it can put your relationship under a lot of strain. This is a time when many marriages break down. The most important thing is to keep communicating. Be ready to adapt and redefine your relationship, and find new goals to work towards as a couple. If you're really struggling, don't be too proud to seek relationship counselling.

Finding love again

Many women find themselves single again in their 40s and 50s, after being divorced or widowed. Entering the dating scene again can be a challenge at this time of life, but many women find unexpected joy in romance and a new relationship. Don't forget that sexually transmitted diseases, including HIV, are on the rise in people in their 40s and 50s. So if you're starting a new relationship, always use condoms, even if you're taking the contraceptive pill.

Over to you!

If you're noticing changes in your sex drive, or physical problems such as vaginal dryness, it's important to keep communicating with your partner about what you both think and feel. Commit together to finding ways around the problem. Can you make changes that will allow both of you to remain happy with your love life? Would simple steps, such as changing your contraceptive or using a lubricant, be sufficient? If you need more help, speak to your doctor about your options. Don't forget to keep using contraceptives until you're certain you can no longer get pregnant.

6

Weight gain after the menopause

If you've found that since becoming menopausal your weight has started creeping up, you're not alone. Many women find it harder to maintain a healthy size after the menopause – and more of a struggle to lose any excess pounds they've gained. Carrying extra weight can dent your self-esteem at just the time when you need a boost. More importantly, being overweight can have a dramatic effect on your health.

Mythbuster

There's nothing you can do about weight gain after 40.
Although it's harder to lose weight with each passing decade, especially after the menopause, many women

successfully slim down in their 40s, 50s, and beyond, by adopting a healthy diet and exercise programme. It just takes a little extra dedication.

Why do you gain weight after the menopause?

Maintaining your weight is all about *Energy In vs Energy Out*. You take in energy (measured in calories) through food and drink. Your body breaks down the food, and the energy is used to maintain all your bodily functions. You also burn energy with every movement you make, from picking up a pen to running a marathon.

You need to consume a certain number of calories a day to keep your weight stable. This depends on your height and build, but for women the average requirement is around 2,000 calories a day. If you consume more calories than you need, and you don't burn them off with exercise, the extra energy is stored as fat. Consume fewer calories than you burn and your body releases the energy stored in fat to make up the difference – and you lose weight.

Your metabolism is the rate at which your body burns energy. Unfortunately, with each passing decade, your metabolism naturally slows down, particularly after the menopause. So to maintain a steady weight, you need to either lower your energy intake or increase your activity levels. Otherwise, the pounds will creep on – and are harder to lose too. Fortunately, there are ways to boost your metabolism.

What people say...

My weight was always fairly steady, and if I did gain a few pounds, I could lose them easily by cutting out cakes and walking more. However, after the menopause, I gained a stone

– and when I tried my usual method of slimming down, I didn't shift a single pound in two months! I realized then that my metabolism had changed and I'd have to alter my approach to maintain my weight. I'm pleased to say I managed it.
Sabina, 49

Why your weight matters
Being overweight or obese raises your risk of heart disease, high blood pressure, stroke, and diabetes. It also increases your likelihood of developing certain cancers, including breast, womb, and colon cancer. Since your risk of many of these conditions increases after the menopause, it's especially important to maintain a healthy weight at this time. If you're overweight, even losing a modest amount can significantly improve your well-being and add years to your life expectancy.

Staying slim will help to keep you mobile, boost your energy levels, and improve your sleep patterns, all of which will make the menopause easier. It can also boost your libido, reduce your risk of stress incontinence, and make you sweat less – which will help with those dreaded hot flushes and night sweats.

How much should you weigh?
You're probably well aware if you've gained weight – it'll show on the scales and in the fit of your clothes. But if you want to know the healthy weight range for your height, try working out your Body Mass Index (BMI). This is used by health professionals to assess whether your weight is putting your health at risk. There are BMI calculators on the internet (in imperial and metric), but if you want to work it out yourself, here's how:

Divide your weight in kilograms by the square of your height in metres. For example, if you weigh 70kg and are 1.75m tall, your BMI is 70 ÷ (1.75 x 1.75), which gives a BMI of 22.9.

Here's how to interpret your BMI:

- Less than 16.5: severely underweight
- 16.5–18.5: underweight
- 18.5–25: healthy weight
- 25–30: overweight
- 30–40: obese
- More than 40: morbidly obese (at risk of potentially life-threatening health problems).

Although BMI is helpful, it's only a guide, and every individual is different. For instance, serious exercisers are often heavier because they have a higher muscle density (muscle weighs more than fat).

The dreaded "muffin top"

Where you store fat on your body also makes a difference to your health. Carrying too much weight around your middle increases your risk of conditions such as heart disease, high blood pressure, type 2 diabetes, and some cancers. Unfortunately, this is precisely the area where many women lay down fat after the menopause, as lower oestrogen levels lead to a change in the distribution of body fat. You have a higher risk of health problems if your waist measures more than 31½ inches (80cm). The risk increases further if your waist is more than 34½ inches (88cm).

Mythbuster

HRT has made me pile on the pounds.
There's no evidence that HRT causes weight gain. It's likely you'd have gained weight at this time whether you were taking HRT or not. With a healthy diet and active lifestyle, you can maintain your size – or even lose excess pounds – while taking HRT. However, if you're convinced your HRT is affecting your body shape, speak to your doctor.

The best way to lose weight
The most effective way to lose weight is to eat a healthy, low-fat diet of no fewer than 1,200 calories a day, and to combine this with an exercise programme to increase your energy output. This doesn't mean never enjoying your favourite treats – it just means practising moderation and "spending" your calories on foods that nourish your body and help it function efficiently.

Aim to lose no more than 1–2lb (0.5–1kg) a week, and never starve yourself. You need to consume a certain number of calories a day to get all the nutrients you require to stay healthy. Besides, losing weight too quickly isn't good for you, and will make you more likely to regain it afterwards. Take it slowly and stick to your plan, and you should see the fat slowly melt away.

Boost your metabolism
Keeping your metabolism ticking along at a good pace, and not allowing it to become sluggish, is essential for maintaining a healthy weight after the menopause. Here are some ways to keep your internal motor functioning efficiently.

Always eat breakfast

It's tempting to skip breakfast to save a few calories, but research shows that people who eat breakfast every day are less likely to be overweight than those who regularly start the day on an empty stomach. That's because your metabolism slows down during the night to conserve energy and get you through the nightly "fast". You need to break that fast ("break-fast") to kick-start your metabolism for the day.

Eat little and often

This will help to keep your metabolism ticking over. It also keeps your blood sugar levels stable, making you less likely to experience an energy dip and reach for a sugary snack. Rather than three large meals a day, eat three small meals and two or three healthy snacks, leaving no longer than three hours between eating.

Don't crash diet

If your energy intake dips too low, your body will go into "starvation mode" and try to hold on to fat stores and lower your metabolism to preserve you through the "famine". When you start eating normally again, your body will lay down fat more quickly, and you may end up heavier than you started.

Stay active

The best way to boost your metabolism is to stay active. If you do at least thirty minutes of moderate exercise, five times a week, you'll find you can be more relaxed about what you eat and the extra pounds will come off more easily. It can also help stabilize your blood sugar levels, which will ease sugar cravings and make it easier to stick to a healthy diet.

Build some muscle

Increasing your muscle mass by exercising with weights (or against your own body weight) means you'll burn more calories per hour, even at rest. It will also make you look more toned and improve your posture. Don't worry about bulking up and developing a masculine physique – bodybuilding takes serious dedication using heavy weights and a high-protein diet, and you can't do it by accident!

What people say...

After twice losing 4st (25kg) and piling it back on again, I was determined not to have to do it again. This time, I continued eating healthily and stayed active, rather than slipping back into being a couch potato. I take our two dogs for long walks every day, and I take my granddaughter swimming twice a week. I have loads of energy and can easily run up the stairs to my third-floor office. I've kept the weight off for three years.
Sandy, 53

The benefits of getting fitter

As well as keeping the flab at bay, exercise boosts your immune system and increases your energy levels. It also improves your quality of sleep, helps maintain mental agility, and releases feel-good hormones to combat stress and improve your mood.

To get the full benefit, your workout should include cardiovascular exercise (which raises your heart rate and makes you breathe harder), resistance training (which uses weights or your own body weight to build muscle strength), and stretching. Don't forget to warm up and cool down to protect your muscles and reduce your likelihood of injury.

Find an activity you enjoy. If going to the gym sounds like a form of torture, how about dancing, cycling, skipping, tennis, swimming, brisk walking, hiking, or heavy gardening? Anything that raises your heart rate and works your muscles will do. If you're not used to exercise, start gently and build up slowly.

Look for ways to be more active in your everyday life – walk rather than drive, take the stairs instead of the lift, and so on. Every exertion will help keep your metabolism ticking over.

Over to you!

If you're struggling to maintain a healthy weight, take an honest look at your diet and activity levels. How can you make improvements? Accept that your changing metabolism means you'll have to alter your lifestyle to maintain your size. If you need to lose weight, decide on a goal and write out a plan for your new, healthy diet and exercise routine. Get the OK from your doctor first if you have a health condition, are very overweight, or haven't exercised for a long time. There's a book in this series called *First Steps out of Weight Problems* – see the **Useful resources** section at the back of this book.

7

Keeping up appearances

Looking good is more of a challenge as we get older and our skin naturally becomes saggy and lacklustre – and trust the menopause to make it that bit harder. Fluctuating hormones can lead to drier skin, thinning hair on the scalp, and an increase in facial and body hair. These changes may be less noticeable if you're taking HRT, but there are other ways to hang on to that youthful glow for as long as possible. It will give you extra confidence to look and feel your best.

Skin-deep

Some experts believe declining oestrogen levels speed up the ageing of your skin. Collagen and elastin – the proteins that keep skin plump and supple – begin to deteriorate, leading to wrinkles and sagging. Loss of moisture in the tissues and membranes makes skin drier. The layer of fat under the surface diminishes, and your skin may become thinner and more easily damaged. Dead skin cells don't shed as efficiently, so you may get dull, dry patches. To cap it all, teenage spots may make a reappearance.

Go for the glow

The jury is out on whether anti-ageing creams really make a difference to lines and wrinkles. Meanwhile, beauty salons are increasingly offering more drastic treatments to hold back the signs of ageing, such as skin peels, dermal fillers, and Botox injections.

However, something as simple as switching to a richer moisturizer and exfoliating twice a week to slough off dead skin cells will help to keep your skin bright and hydrated. Be gentle with your delicate eye area, and don't neglect your neck and hands, which can become crêpey and give away your age.

Staying out of the sun and using a high-SPF sunblock both play a big part in holding back the years, as UV rays are the main offender for damaging the collagen in your skin. Giving up smoking and not drinking too much alcohol or caffeine will also keep you looking youthful for longer. Exercise boosts blood flow to your skin, helping to deliver nutrients and remove waste matter to make your complexion clearer and more glowing.

A healthy diet that's rich in antioxidants (such as vitamins A, C, and E) will feed your skin. Foods rich in omega-3 and omega-6 essential fatty acids, such as olive oil, nuts, seeds, and oily fish, help to protect your skin from moisture loss. Drink plenty of water to hydrate your skin from the inside and keep it plump and healthy.

Flush-proof your make-up

If your make-up ends up sliding off your face when you have hot flushes, don't panic. A mattifying primer under your make-up (or on its own) will keep oil levels down and help your make-up stay put. Choose matte make-up formulations to help keep your face in place. If you're really struggling, ask at a make-up counter about brands designed for hot climates or stage lighting.

Mythbuster

More make-up will make me look younger.

Heavy make-up can actually be ageing, as foundation and powder settle in fine lines and accentuate them. A lighter foundation or tinted moisturizer can work better for older skin, and a cream blusher may look less caked-on than a powder. A light-reflecting base – on its own or under foundation – can work wonders, giving you a glow and minimizing wrinkles. It's a good idea to revamp your make-up bag from time to time, especially if you've used the same colours for years – your natural skin tone fades over time, so subtler colours are more flattering.

Hair today, gone tomorrow

Greying hair has nothing to do with hormonal changes, but around a third of women experience thinning or receding hair after the menopause. This is because hair follicles are receptive to hormones, and as oestrogen declines, the influence of androgens ("male" hormones) becomes stronger, so you develop a mild form of male pattern baldness. Hair also grows more slowly and each hair becomes more slender. Your hair may become drier and duller, due to the oil glands in your scalp becoming less active.

Maintain your crowning glory

Hair loss is notoriously difficult to prevent, although some women find supplements containing iron, zinc, and B vitamins help. However, disguising the thinning areas can be as simple as choosing a new hairstyle. Updating your look will give you a confidence boost too. Have a chat with your hairdresser about what styles may suit you and draw attention away from problem areas.

Richer, more moisturizing shampoos, regular hot oil treatments, and anti-frizz serums can all help to rehydrate dry hair, making it look fuller and healthier. Regular trims will help keep it in good condition.

Mythbuster

Colouring my grey hair will hold back the years.
Grey hair can be ageing – but as skin tone fades with age, darker hair can look harsh and less flattering, and blonde can look brassy. Brunettes should go for a colour a few shades lighter than their original natural colour. Lighter shades won't show grey regrowth as much, either. Blondes should try more honey-coloured shades. On the other hand, many women embrace their grey and can look very elegant.

What people say...

Since the menopause, my hair has thinned and receded slightly on each side. It isn't something that worries me a great deal, but I keep my hair longer where it's receding and brush it carefully to avoid the thin patches showing. I've been colouring my grey for many years, but I recently started using a lighter shade to flatter my changing skin tone, which I probably should have done years ago. My face has become more marked with age spots, although I don't know if that's due to the menopause or just getting older. I once tried a lightening cream to fade them, which didn't work, so now I use a light foundation to disguise them.

Josephine, 66

Facing up to unwanted hair

To add insult to injury, just as you're losing the hair on your head, you may find you're gaining it on your face and body. Again, this is due to the changing balance between "male" and "female" hormones in your body.

Beat the beard

There isn't much you can do to prevent those whiskers sprouting from your chin, upper lip, and other less attractive places, but there are plenty of ways to deal with them. If there are only a few, plucking them with tweezers will probably be sufficient. Otherwise, you can opt for bleaching, depilatory (hair removal) cream, or waxing – at home or in a salon.

For a permanent solution, try electrolysis, where a hair-thin metal probe is inserted into each hair follicle and a small electrical current passed through it to kill the root. Six or more sessions may be required.

Alternatively, laser hair removal or intense pulsed light (IPL) can quickly and permanently destroy large areas of hair follicles. They're more expensive than electrolysis and may take six or more sessions to work, but they're the most effective hair removal techniques currently available. They work best on people with dark hair and pale skin. Ask your local salon for advice.

What people say...

I have dark hair, thanks to my Mediterranean background, and I've always battled with unwanted face and body hair. However, after I started the menopause, I noticed a definite increase in coarse hairs sprouting from my chin, cheeks, upper lip, and nipples. I was fighting a losing battle with waxing and bleaching at home, and always carried tweezers in case I caught sight of them in a mirror! Electrolysis didn't really do the trick – new hairs were appearing faster than the beautician could "zap" them. In the end, I opted for IPL. It wasn't cheap, but after eight sessions, the hairs were all gone – hopefully for good.
Carolina, 47

Over to you!

If you're noticing changes in your skin and hair, take time to review your beauty routine and make some changes. Would a richer moisturizer or lighter foundation work better with your changing skin? Should you update your hairstyle or colour? If you're feeling down about how you look, consider treating yourself to a visit to the beauty salon or hairdresser to boost your confidence. If you're struggling with unwanted facial or body hair, do some research into the best methods for keeping it at bay. However, if your facial hair seems unusually coarse, speak to your doctor, as it could be caused by a more serious hormonal imbalance.

8

Protecting your future health

Although the menopause itself isn't a medical condition, declining oestrogen levels can increase your risk of other serious diseases, including osteoporosis and heart disease. Your likelihood of developing hormone-related cancers, such as breast cancer, also increases. However, there are ways to lower your risk – and the earlier you take action, the more effective it will be.

Boning up

Osteoporosis (brittle bones) is a thinning of the bone tissue. This leads to bones becoming weak and fragile, and more vulnerable to breaks and fractures. Many people have no idea they have osteoporosis until their first broken bone. In advanced cases, even a little knock, cough, or sneeze can lead to a fracture. It can be very disabling, making it difficult to enjoy a normal life.

The most common fractures are of the wrist, hip, and vertebrae (spine bones). Small fractures in the spine can lead to stooping and chronic back pain. A fracture of a major bone such as the hip can lead to permanent disability or indirectly to death – around 30 per cent of people over 75 who break a hip will die within a year, as lack of mobility increases their risk of respiratory conditions and other problems.

The oestrogen connection

Until the age of around 30, a healthy body is actively laying down calcium and building bone density. From about 35 onwards, you naturally start losing bone density. However, the decline of oestrogen after the menopause rapidly accelerates bone loss, as sex hormones play a major part in helping your body absorb calcium and remodel your bones. Post-menopausal women are the most common sufferers of osteoporosis – nearly half of all women over 50 suffer a fracture, mainly due to weakened bones. You're at greater risk if you have an early menopause (or started your periods late).

Mythbuster

It's too late to do anything for my bones.
It's harder for your body to lay down calcium after the age of about 35, so the sooner you begin taking steps to protect and build up your bones, the better. However, the same methods you use to build up your bones will also

help to slow down their loss, so it's never too late to start looking after your skeleton.

Protect your bones

Weight-bearing exercise, undertaken regularly, is known to help build up bone tissue, but don't worry, this doesn't mean lifting weights in the gym. Weight-bearing exercise is any activity that involves supporting your own body weight – try brisk walking, running, dancing, aerobics, or tennis. Swimming and cycling don't count as weight-bearing, as the water or bicycle carries the weight for you.

Eating plenty of calcium-rich foods is vital for building and maintaining bones. Even young women can develop osteoporosis if they don't consume enough calcium (for instance, in cases of anorexia), leading to irreversible weakening of their bones. Foods that are rich in calcium include dairy products (milk, cheese, yogurt), dried fruit, tofu, and green leafy vegetables such as broccoli. If you struggle to get enough calcium in your diet – for instance, if you're dairy-intolerant or vegan – try eating calcium-enriched foods such as breads, cereals, orange juice, and soya products. You can also take a calcium supplement (check with your doctor first).

For calcium to be properly absorbed, you also need good levels of vitamin D. This is found in fish oils, eggs, brown rice, and lentils, and the body produces its own vitamin D in the presence of sunlight. Many calcium supplements include vitamin D to aid absorption, and studies have shown that a daily calcium and vitamin D supplement can reduce your risk of a hip fracture by over 20 per cent. Good levels of phosphorus and magnesium also encourage calcium absorption.

Giving up smoking and keeping your alcohol intake low will also help to protect your bones. Avoid drinking tea and coffee with meals, as this interferes with the absorption of nutrients from food. Some experts believe carbonated (fizzy) drinks increase bone loss, but the jury's currently out on this.

What people say...

I suffered several small fractures and my back was often sore, so my doctor referred me for a bone density scan. It showed I had advanced bone thinning in my hips and spine. I was shocked as I'd always eaten well and exercised, and there was no family history of osteoporosis. I was told it may be connected to an emergency hysterectomy I'd had after a difficult birth, which led to premature menopause at age 37. I now take medication to help prevent further bone loss. I also eat plenty of calcium-rich foods and take a calcium supplement, and I stay active with walking and gardening. My bone density has increased slightly and I'm still enjoying life.
Penny, 59

Over to you!

If you have a family history of osteoporosis, or are at high risk for other reasons, such as being underweight, having a history of eating disorders, early menopause, or malabsorption conditions (such as coeliac disease or Crohn's disease), ask your doctor for a bone density scan. If you're diagnosed with osteoporosis, there are a number of medications to help slow down the deterioration. HRT also offers some protection by delaying the decline of oestrogen in your body.

Take heart

Coronary heart disease involves the narrowing of blood vessels that supply blood and oxygen to the heart. Thickening and hardening of the arteries (atherosclerosis) can lead to a restriction in blood flow, starving the heart of oxygen and causing a heart attack (when part of the heart muscle is damaged or dies). Angina is where an artery is narrowed, but not totally blocked off, causing pain in the chest, neck, arm, shoulder, or jaw. If blood flow to the brain is restricted, it can lead to a stroke or death.

There are a number of risk factors for heart disease, including a high-fat diet, lack of exercise, stress, smoking, drinking too much alcohol, being overweight, high blood pressure, high cholesterol levels, and a genetic predisposition.

Mythbuster

Heart disease is a man's problem.

It's true that more men than women develop heart disease. However, heart attack is the leading cause of death in both men and women – and after the menopause, women catch up quite a bit in the heart disease stakes. Furthermore, if a woman has a heart attack, she's more likely than a man to die from it, partly because the warning signs often aren't as obvious in women.

The oestrogen connection

Oestrogen offers significant protection for the heart – which is partly why, up to the age of around 50, men are more likely to have a heart attack or stroke than women. Oestrogen helps to dilate the blood vessels, stops blood clotting too readily, and lowers "bad" cholesterol. All this gives women a major advantage – until their oestrogen levels start dropping during the menopause.

HRT and your heart

Taking HRT slightly increases your risk of abnormal blood clotting and high blood pressure – and, in turn, your likelihood of having a stroke or heart attack. So if you have a history (or family history) of heart disease, or are at high risk for other reasons, you may not be suitable for HRT. However, for most people, the risks of HRT are low and are outweighed by the benefits.

Protect your heart

To lower your risk of heart disease, eat a low-fat diet, rich in fruit, vegetables, and wholegrains (such as wholemeal bread, wholewheat pasta, and brown rice). Avoid saturated fats and salt (mostly in processed foods), cut back on red meat, and eat oily fish (such as sardines, herring, salmon, and tuna) twice a week.

Don't smoke, and limit yourself to one alcoholic drink a day. Get plenty of exercise (at least thirty minutes, five times a week) and keep your weight within a healthy range. Getting enough sleep and keeping your stress levels

 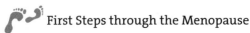

as low as possible have also been shown to reduce your risk of heart problems.

Have your blood pressure and cholesterol checked regularly, and take steps to lower them if they're too high. Your doctor may prescribe medications to help with this. If you already have heart disease, your doctor may give you drugs to reduce your chances of a heart attack or stroke.

What people say...

I used to work long hours and lived on coffee, stress, and smoking – but because there's no family history of heart disease and I wasn't overweight, it didn't occur to me that I was at risk. Four years ago, aged 51, I had a heart attack and had to have two stents fitted in a blood vessel going into my heart. I couldn't believe it was happening to me. After cardiac rehab, I quit smoking and began making an effort to eat well and exercise. My cholesterol is now at a healthy level, and I feel and look much better. I'm going to stick to my new lifestyle and see my grandchildren grow up.
Cathy, 55

Over to you!

If you're at risk of heart disease, try to improve your lifestyle to reduce your chances of developing problems. Ideally, you'd do this before the menopause, but it's never too late to improve your heart health, and losing even a modest amount of weight can make a big difference. If you have a history (or family history) of heart problems or stroke, consider whether HRT is a wise option for you – your doctor may not prescribe it for you anyway. Seek medical help immediately if you experience any unexpected shortness of breath; pain in the chest, arm, or jaw; a swollen, painful leg; or any loss of movement, especially on one side.

Breast cancer and other hormone-related cancers

The menopause isn't believed to be a specific risk factor for cancers, but most cancers increase in women after the age of 50, and oestrogen plays a part in some of them. HRT can also have an effect.

Breast cancer is the most common cancer in women, and sex hormones can play a role in its development. The earlier you start menstruating, and the later you have your menopause – in other words, the longer you have periods – the greater your risk. Having children before the age of 30 lowers your likelihood of getting breast cancer, as does breastfeeding. Taking the contraceptive pill slightly elevates your risk, but it gradually returns to normal after you stop taking it.

Similarly, the chance of developing ovarian cancer and endometrial cancer (cancer of the womb lining) increases after the age of 50, and is more common in women who've never been pregnant or breastfed. Risk also increases with early puberty and late menopause. However, taking the contraceptive pill actually lowers your risk of these cancers.

Other risk factors for cancer include family history or genetic predisposition, an unhealthy diet, being overweight, not exercising regularly, smoking, and drinking too much alcohol.

If you develop cancer before the menopause, chemotherapy can cause premature menopause. You can read more about that in Chapter 9.

I'm too young to get cancer.

Although your chance of developing all kinds of cancers, including "female" cancers, increases with age, you can get cancer at any age. That's why it's important to stay healthy, be vigilant about self-examination and screening, and see your doctor if you develop any unusual symptoms.

HRT and cancer

Taking HRT can very slightly raise your risk of some cancers, including breast, endometrial, and ovarian cancer – and the longer you take it, the greater your risk. However, it depends on the kind of HRT you're taking (oestrogen-only or combined), and after you stop taking it, your risk slowly returns to normal. If you have any history (or family history) of hormone-related cancers, you may not be considered suitable for HRT, so discuss this with your doctor. You can learn more about HRT and cancer in Chapter 2.

Over to you!

Lower your cancer risk now by adopting a healthy, low-fat diet including plenty of fruit and vegetables. Lose weight if you need to, and start exercising regularly. If you smoke, giving up will lower your risk, as will keeping down your alcohol intake. Cancer survival rates depend very much on early diagnosis, so practise self-examination (of breasts) regularly, and take advantage of all screening programmes offered to you.

9

Premature menopause

A premature menopause is usually defined as one that occurs before the age of 45 (or 40, depending on who you ask). Also known as "premature ovarian failure", it affects around 1 per cent of women under the age of 40; and 1 in 1,000 under the age of 30. It's even possible to go through the menopause in your teens, but this is very rare, affecting just one in 10,000 women.

Premature menopause happens for a number of reasons. For some women, the hormone system stops functioning early due to a disease or genetic abnormality. In other cases, it's caused by medical treatments such as chemotherapy or hysterectomy.

Women who have an early menopause are usually offered HRT and/or other treatments to relieve symptoms. You can continue taking HRT for longer than the usual five years, as the benefits outweigh any potential risks.

However, there are other issues to contend with, such as loss of fertility and how a woman feels about her sexuality and femininity.

What causes premature menopause?

When an early menopause occurs "naturally" ("primary" premature ovarian failure), there's often no obvious cause. It's believed that in around 5 per cent of cases, there's a genetic link, so you may find other women in your family have had the same experience.

In some cases, it can be due to an enzyme deficiency interfering with oestrogen production. Or it can be a side effect of an autoimmune disease, such as thyroid disease, rheumatoid arthritis, or diabetes, when the body's immune system attacks its own tissues (in this case, the ovaries). Very rarely, premature ovarian failure can be the result of an infection such as tuberculosis, mumps, malaria, or chickenpox.

Chromosomal abnormalities, such as Down's syndrome, Turner's syndrome, or a defect of the X (female) chromosome, will usually lead to early menopause. The same is true of "intersex" conditions, such as androgen insensitivity syndrome (where the person is genetically male but presents as female), or Mayer-Rokitansky-Küster-Hauser syndrome (where the uterus and vagina are underdeveloped or absent). However, these conditions are extremely rare.

Mythbuster

If my periods stop early, it must mean premature menopause.

Periods can stop at any age for many reasons, including being underweight. If you're having menopausal symptoms or unusual bleeding patterns before the age of 40, your doctor will want to run tests for conditions such as thyroid disease or cervical cancer, which can produce similar symptoms. So don't delay in seeking medical advice.

Medical menopause

Some women go through an early menopause after chemotherapy to treat cancer (not necessarily in the reproductive organs). Radiotherapy in the ovary area can have a similar effect. The risk of this "secondary" premature ovarian failure depends on the type of treatment and the age of the patient – younger (teenage) women tend to tolerate it better.

Chemotherapy is designed to destroy rapidly dividing cancer cells. Unfortunately, it often damages healthy cells too, particularly rapidly dividing ones – which is why hair follicles, bone marrow, and ovaries are commonly affected. Healthy cells often repair themselves in the long run, but ovaries don't always recover.

If you're facing chemotherapy or radiotherapy, ask your specialist about the risk to your fertility, and the possibility of freezing your eggs for future IVF or surrogacy.

Surgical menopause

The removal of your uterus (hysterectomy) can lead to an early menopause. If the ovaries are removed as well, there'll be an immediate "surgical" menopause, as oestrogen is no longer being manufactured by the ovaries. This kind of surgery may be needed for ovarian cancer, cysts, and endometriosis (where cells from the womb lining migrate elsewhere in the body, commonly the ovaries). Menopausal symptoms can kick in quickly, while you're still recovering from the operation.

If you're facing this kind of surgery, ask your surgeon exactly what will be removed, what can safely be left, and what the effects will be. Again, you may want to ask about freezing your eggs for future use.

Facing infertility

The major issue for younger women going through the menopause is the end of reproductive potential. This can be very difficult to come to terms with, even if you already have a family, and it can be devastating if you've not yet had children.

However, premature menopause doesn't necessarily mean you'll never have a family – it may just require some lateral thinking. If you've had a chance to freeze your eggs and you still have your uterus, you may be able to have IVF. If you're unable to use your own eggs, you may be able to use eggs from a donor, fertilized with your partner's sperm.

Another option is surrogacy – where another woman carries a child for you, using eggs that are yours, hers, or donated. However, egg donors and surrogates are hard to find, and it's a tough process that often ends in disappointment, so you should talk it through carefully with your partner before proceeding.

Many couples create their longed-for family through adoption. This can be a demanding but deeply satisfying experience, with the added joy of giving a loving home to a child who needs one.

Finally, some women settle on being "positively childless", making the most of the freedom and benefits they can enjoy by not being responsible for young children.

What people say...
I suffered terribly with endometriosis, spending three weeks a month tired and in pain, although I was fortunate enough to have two children. At 35, it became too much and I had a full hysterectomy, including one ovary. I immediately went into menopause – hot flushes, loss of sex drive, and mood swings. HRT sorted out my physical symptoms, but it was hard to accept I'd have no more children, as I'd always wanted a large family. I don't regret the surgery, though, as I feel stronger, healthier, and better able to look after my children.
Rachel, 39

Changing self-image

An early menopause can have a profound effect on how you view yourself and your sexuality. Many women feel less feminine, less attractive, and "less of a woman". Unsurprisingly, premature ovarian failure is often associated with depression – and it's worse if you're coping with it in isolation. Talking to a counsellor or other women going through similar experiences can be invaluable in helping you come to terms with it.

The effect on your sex life can also be tough to cope with at a time when you expect to be at your sexual peak and may be at a relatively early stage in a relationship. Turn to Chapter 5 for ways to keep your sex life on track.

What people say...

At 32, I was diagnosed with Burkitt's lymphoma and had four rounds of chemotherapy. Thankfully, I was cured of the lymphoma, but then came the migraines, hot flushes, and dryness "down below", and it was clear I was going through the menopause. It really affected how feminine I felt, even though my husband did all he could to make me feel better. HRT deals with the physical symptoms, but I found infertility extremely hard to bear, and went through a period of mourning for the babies I'd never have. However, we now have a wonderful six-month-old son through surrogacy, and I'm in a happy stage of life.
Leah, 39

Long-term health risks

Early menopause puts you at greater risk of health conditions associated with a decline in oestrogen – primarily osteoporosis and heart disease. HRT gives extra protection, and you may also be offered calcium tablets to protect your bones. However, it's also wise to make lifestyle changes to lower your risk (see Chapter 8).

Over to you!

If you're under 45 and are experiencing menopausal symptoms or unusual bleeding patterns, book an appointment with your doctor. They can investigate the possibility of other conditions that cause similar symptoms, or confirm you're having an early menopause. You may be referred to a specialist. For emotional support, consider joining an organization such as the Daisy Network, where you can learn more about what's happening in your body and chat to other women going through the same thing. See the **Useful resources** section at the back of this book.

10

The best years of your life

As the menopause approaches, you may wonder if it heralds the end of life as you know it, with little more to look forward to than the descent into old age, ill health, and dependency. So you'll be pleasantly surprised to discover the best may be yet to come.

Women today can expect to live a third or more of their lives after the menopause, and you should expect to make the most of it. Although you may experience symptoms for some time after your final period, your hormones will eventually settle down, and you can enjoy the freedom of life without periods and contraception. The post-menopausal years can be a time of opportunity and self-discovery, when you can concentrate on yourself for a change and discover new interests and passions.

What people say...
Since the hot flushes and sleepless nights have settled down and I've come out the other side, I've found it's a good time. Things feel as if they've fitted into place emotionally. I feel wiser and more confident about who I am, and I have more energy than before. And now our children have left home, my husband and I can indulge our love of hiking every weekend.
Jessie, 55

New-found freedom

One of the things women enjoy most after the menopause is freedom from periods – and the hassle, pain, and mood swings that can go with them. Because your hormones no longer go through a cycle of rising and falling in preparation for a potential pregnancy, you can forget the PMS, tiredness, and depression you may have experienced every month for decades. Plus there's no more taking painkillers, worrying about falling pregnant, or planning events and holidays around heavy periods.

What people say...
The end of periods is just great! No more worrying about what to wear, carrying tampons, or the embarrassment of having to beg a sanitary towel from someone you hardly know if you're caught short. Now I can do what I like, when I like – sports, swimming, and hiking in the hills. It's amazing how quickly you forget what a nuisance periods were – goodbye and good riddance! Plus, I can blame the menopause for getting plump – it wasn't all those cream cakes and chocolate bars after all!
Judy, 62

I'll never have sex again.

Although the menopause can cause lower libido and sexual difficulties, many women find they want and enjoy sex as much or even more after the menopause and, with a few adjustments, go on enjoying it into old age. No longer having to worry about contraception, unwanted pregnancy, or disturbing other family members in the house can release you to be more spontaneous, uninhibited, and confident – so for many couples it's a new beginning. It's also a time when many women start new and exciting relationships after divorce or being widowed. Far from being the end, you may be looking forward to many more years of sexual pleasure.

Indulge yourself

If you have more time on your hands – and maybe a little more disposable cash as the mortgage is paid off and children leave home – take the opportunity to indulge yourself. If you're worried about your changing image, set aside time to reassess your style and wardrobe, and invest in some flattering new clothes. Enjoy being pampered at the beauty salon, have your hair done regularly, and invest in some gorgeous new underwear. It'll all help you look and feel your best. It may even give your relationship a boost, or make you feel more confident about meeting a new partner.

What people say...

The menopause isn't a time I like to look back on, but I'm through it now and in a different place. I'm free from hormonal cycles, PMS, and the pain of endometriosis. I walk past the sanitary towels in the supermarket without a backward glance. Plus I have more energy and get more done.

Margaret, 49

It's time for you

Mid-life can be a wonderful time for women to rediscover themselves. As children fly the nest to set up their own homes, and retirement beckons for you and your partner, you may have a freedom you've never experienced before.

After the menopause, lower levels of oestrogen and oxytocin (the "love hormone") may mean you become less emotional and feel less compelled to take a mothering or nurturing role towards others. That doesn't mean you'll become selfish or unloving, but you may be able to focus more on your own desires and ambitions and develop new interests – or revive those that had to go on the back burner while you raised your family.

Many women feel they have the wisdom and confidence to reinvent themselves, go back to studying, travel the world, or begin a new business. Look after yourself so you stay healthy, and the sky is the limit.

What people say...

I had very few symptoms during the menopause, and no weight gain at all. In fact, I've lost a few pounds – perhaps due to rediscovering my passion for horses and riding, which keeps me busy, active, and out in the fresh air. I no longer have the monthly depression, water retention, and inconvenient bleeding I had before. The menopause really hasn't been the misery I expected.

Lorna, 59

Over to you!

Take time to review what you want from your life. Are you happy in your job, or would this be a good time to make changes or try something new? If retirement is on the horizon for you and your partner, how do you plan to use your time? Are there hobbies you've always wanted to try, interests you'd like to develop, or subjects you want to study? Are there friends you'd like to spend more time with, or places you want to visit? Is your relationship feeling stale, and if so, how can you breathe new life into it? Make a plan and start taking action to shake things up, get out of your rut, and begin an exciting new phase in your life.

For the family

The menopause is a natural transition in every woman's life, but while some sail through it without difficulties, for others it's a tough time. Not only does a woman have to contend with physical changes, but she can also be affected mentally and emotionally. This is thanks not only to fluctuating hormones but also to having to come to terms with the end of fertility, the ageing process, and facing a new stage in her life.

As your loved one goes through this major life event, her experiences are likely to affect the whole family. You might struggle to know how to support her as she struggles with physical symptoms such as hot flushes and urinary infections. You may be bewildered by changes in her mood and temperament. If you're her partner, you may find your sex life affected by her waning libido and painful intercourse.

Expect change
It can be puzzling when someone you've known a long time starts behaving in ways that seem out of character and irrational, and it may be tempting to tell her to pull herself together. However, it's essential to recognize that

your loved one is dealing with many challenges, both physical and emotional, and these are bound to affect her outlook.

It will help if you have some understanding of the changes taking place in her body and how these may affect her, so take time to educate yourself on the menopause. Reading this book is a good place to start. She'll appreciate you caring enough to take an interest.

Support her

Your family member may have to make decisions about how to deal with her symptoms. She might want to explore the option of HRT, or perhaps she's more comfortable taking the "natural" route. Discovering what works best for her may be a process of trial and error. It will help if you're willing to listen and talk through the different approaches as she weighs up her options, and try to be supportive of her decisions. She may want you to accompany her to doctor's appointments for moral support or so you can better understand what she's going through.

It will help your loved one if you're willing to lighten the load by taking on more chores at home. She may be exhausted from night sweats and sleepless nights, or struggling with depression and irritability. This may coincide with a time when she's under extra strain, caring for children or elderly parents. Having time to rest will help to reduce her stress levels and, in turn, her physical and emotional symptoms. If she can spend more time looking after herself – exercising, exploring complementary therapies, or caring for her physical appearance – the whole family will benefit.

Be flexible

Because this is a time of change, not just for your loved one but also for the entire family, taking a flexible approach will help. For instance, be willing to adapt your eating habits so she can improve her diet to protect her future health. Or start being more active as a family, such as going walking or cycling together, to increase her fitness levels.

If you're her partner, and she's struggling with insomnia and night sweats, it will help if you're willing to consider new sleeping arrangements. Separate mattresses, beds, or even rooms can make all the difference to getting a decent night's sleep – for you as well as her. It doesn't have to mean the end of sex or affection, but you may have to be more creative about it.

On the other hand, your sex life may be affected by changes in your partner's body, and it will help to be flexible about that too. She may have to change her contraceptive methods. Sex might become painful, so a gentler approach with less emphasis on intercourse may help. Her libido may drop, which could be difficult for you to cope with. The important thing is to keep communicating and looking for compromises.

If you're still hoping to have children and the menopause has arrived sooner than expected, this will be an extra source of stress and grief for you and your partner. Being positive about exploring other means of having a family – such as adoption, IVF, or egg donation – will help to lessen her distress.

Reassure her

This can be a tumultuous time in a woman's life, and your family member may feel vulnerable. She may feel the menopause has robbed her of something fundamental about her femininity and womanhood, especially if she's experiencing it prematurely. She may go through a period of mourning. Being there to give her a reassuring hug will help.

Your loved one may be feeling less attractive as she struggles with weight gain, dry skin, and receding hair. If you're her partner, assuring her you still find her desirable and consider her a "complete woman" will help. Perhaps you could treat her to a trip to the beauty salon or a flattering new outfit to boost her self-esteem.

Most of all, knowing her family members understand what she's going through and are supporting her will help your loved one through to the other side. It won't last for ever – her hormones will even out and you can all move on to a new, positive stage of life.

Useful resources

General menopause information

- Read *Menopause for Dummies* by Dr Sarah Brewer, Marcia L. Jones and Dr Theresa Eichenwald (John Wiley & Sons, 2007)

- Read *Menopause: The Guide for Real Women* by Caroline Carr (White Ladder, 2009)

For information and support

- www.menopausematters.co.uk

- www.womens-health-concern.org

- www.simplyhormones.com

- www.menopause.org.uk

For clinical information relating to your country

- **UK:** British Menopause Society – www.thebms.org.uk

- **USA:** North American Menopause Society – www.menopause.org

- **Canada:** Society of Obstetricians and Gynaecologists of Canada – www.menopauseandu.ca

- **Australia:** Australasian Menopause Society – www.menopause.org.au

- **New Zealand:** NZ Menopause Institute – www.nzmenopause.co.nz

- **South Africa:** South African Menopause Society – www.samenopausesociety.co.za

Natural health and complementary therapies

- Read *Natural Solutions to Menopause* by Marilyn Glenville (Rodale, 2011)

- Read *Your Change, Your Choice* by Michael Dooley and Sarah Stacey (Mobius, 2006)

- For sleep sprays, sleep pillows, and aromatherapy products for the menopause, visit: www.innerscents.co.uk

To find a complementary medicine practitioner in your country

- **UK:** Institute for Complementary and Natural Medicine – www.icnm.org.uk

- **USA:** National Center for Complementary and Alternative Medicine – www.nccam.nih.gov

- **Canada:** Natural Healthcare Canada – www.naturalhealthcare.ca
Alternative and Integrative Medical Society – www.aims.ubc.ca

 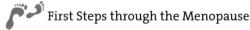

- **Australia and New Zealand:** Australasian Integrative Medicine Association – www.aima.net.au

- **South Africa:** South African Society of Integrative Medicine – www.integrativemedicine.co.za

Premature menopause

- **International:** International Premature Ovarian Failure Association – www.pofsupport.org

- **UK:** The Daisy Network – www.daisynetwork.org.uk

- **Australia:** Australian Early Menopause Network – www.aemn.com.au

- **New Zealand:** NZ Early Menopause Support Group – www.earlymenopause.org.nz

Surrogacy and egg donation

- **UK:** COTS (Childlessness Overcome Through Surrogacy) – www.surrogacy.org.uk
Donor Conception Network – www.donor-conception-network.org

- **Canada:** Surrogacy in Canada Online – www.surrogacy.ca

- **Australia:** Surrogacy Australia – www.surrogacyaustralia.org

- **New Zealand:** NZ Surrogacy – www.nz-surrogacy.com

- **South Africa:** Surrogacy Advisory Group – www.surrogacy.co.za

Mental health

For help with anxiety and depression, and contact information for support organizations around the world, read *First Steps out of Anxiety* by Kate Middleton (Lion Hudson, 2010) and *First Steps out of Depression* by Sue Atkinson (Lion Hudson, 2010).

Weight control

For advice on losing and maintaining your weight, including online resources and contact information for slimming clubs around the world, read *First Steps out of Weight Problems* by Catherine Francis (Lion Hudson, 2012).

Also currently available in the "First Steps" series:

First Steps out of Anxiety
Dr Kate Middleton

First Steps through Bereavement
Sue Mayfield

First Steps out of Depression
Sue Atkinson

First Steps out of Eating Disorders
Dr Kate Middleton
and Jane Smith

First Steps out of Problem Drinking
John McMahon

First Steps out of Problem Gambling
Lisa Mills and Joanna Hughes

First Steps through Separation and Divorce
Penny Rich

First Steps out of Weight Problems
Catherine Francis

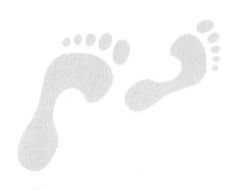